Cued Articulation
Consonants and Vowels
Revised edition

Jane Passy

ACER Press

First published 1990
This edition published 2010
by ACER Press, an imprint of
Australian Council *for* Educational Research Ltd
19 Prospect Hill Road, Camberwell
Victoria, 3124, Australia
www.acerpress.com.au
sales@acer.edu.au

Reprinted 2011, 2013, 2014 (twice), 2015, 2016

Edited by Elisa Webb
Cover and text design by ACER Project Publishing
Printed in Australia by McPherson's Printing Group

National Library of Australia Cataloguing-in-Publication data:

Author: Passy, Jane

Title: Cued Articulation: Consonants and Vowels/Jane Passy

Edition: Rev. ed.

ISBN: 9780864318466 (pbk.)

Subjects: English language - Phonetics
                                 English language - Phonemics
                                 Sound symbolism

Other Authors/Contributors: Australian Council for Educational Research

Dewey Number: 421.5

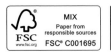

For Luke, who inspired me

to think of different ways of doing things.

About the author

Jane Passy qualified from the Oldrey Fleming School of Speech Therapy, London in 1957. She has worked in many settings, both educational and medical, in England, India and Australia. Her experience with phonetics stood her in good stead when she taught Spoken English to children and young adults from all over Asia while living in India from 1959 until 1967. Her interest in speech and language-disordered children, and the enormous difficulty they have in recalling and producing meaningful speech sounds, inspired her to devise a system of hand cues and colour codes which she called *Cued Articulation*.

Jane retired from clinical practice in 1992, and promoted the *Cued Articulation* system throughout the United Kingdom, Ireland and South Africa.

This new format of the system in colour, with the consonants and vowels in one book, is the sixth publication since it was devised in the late 1970s. The new face in this production is her daughter Hilary.

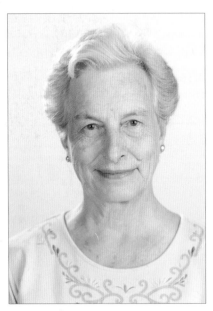

Jane Passy

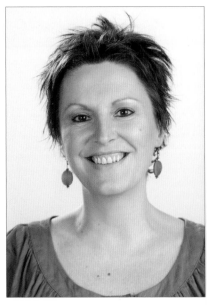

Hilary Phelan

Contents

About the author   *iv*

Cued Articulation *2*

The organs of speech   *2*

The consonants *4*

Consonant table   *7*

List of consonants   *9*

The vowels *37*

Diphthongs   *38*

Triphthongs   *38*

The vowel sounds of Standard English   *40*

List of vowels   *43*

Cued Articulation

The idea of *Cued Articulation* is to simplify what is very difficult to some people, viz. the organisation and pronunciation of spoken English.

This book describes a method of cueing the consonants and vowels, which make up the sounds of Standard English, by using simple hand signs, and it is hoped it will assist all those who find it difficult to remember how to produce these sounds. The method also helps those who have a poor grasp of spelling by the colour coding of the consonant sounds.

The technique has proved to be successful, and has become an excellent educational tool for speech and language therapists, primary teachers, reading recovery teachers, migrant teachers, teachers' aides, visiting teachers of the hearing impaired, and those who have English as a second language.

The organs of speech

The diagram opposite represents the speech organs. Imagine looking into the face from the side. The shape of the nasal and oral cavity is changed by the way the different organs of speech are moved and altered, and the way the air from the lungs is thus hindered in its passage through the mouth or nose.

For instance when the lips come together and the air is stopped behind them and then released, a / p / sound is heard. This is known as a bi-labial plosive. In the case of the / p / sound vocal cords do not vibrate, therefore, there is no sound from the vocal cords, so the / p / is known in phonetic terms as a voiceless bi-labial plosive. In the case of the / b / sound the lips are placed, and the air is stopped in the same manner as for the / p / sound but in the case of the / b / sound the vocal cords do vibrate, so / b / is called a voiced bi-labial plosive. All the consonants are charted on page 7 as to where they are made and how they are made and whether they are voiced or voiceless.

As you come to learn the cues you will realise why *Cued Articulation* is such a useful teaching tool. Each cue gives so much information with so little effort. One simple hand sign shows where, and how, a sound is made and whether that sound is voiced or voiceless.

Organs of speech

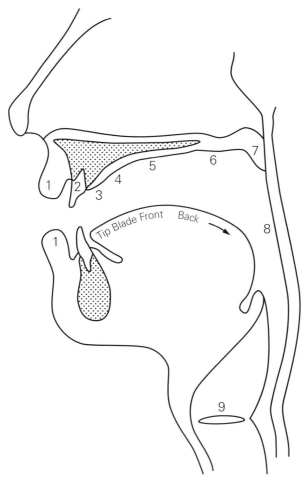

1. Lips (labial)
2. Teeth (dental)
3. Alveolar ridge (alveolar)
4. Hard palate (pre-palatal)
5. Hard palate (palatal)
6. Soft palate (velar)
7. Uvula (uvular)
8. Pharynx (pharyngeal)
9. Glottis (glottal)

The consonants

The hand movements used are logical. Each hand sign represents one phoneme (speech sound). The method in which the fingers are moved indicates whether the phoneme is a plosive (the air is actually stopped and then released to make the sound), a continuant (where the air is allowed to pass through the mouth without obstruction), or an affricate (a combination of the two). The position of the hand indicates whether the phoneme is a front, back or nasal sound. The shape of the hand suggests lip and tongue positions and movements. The number of fingers used indicates whether the phoneme is to be voiced or voiceless; when one finger is used the phoneme is voiceless and when two fingers are used the phoneme is voiced. Thus manner, placement and voicing of each phoneme is indicated by one simple movement of the hand.

The phonemes are set out in their phonological groupings, not in alphabetical order. This makes it easier to see how each of the consonants are related to each other especially when the colour coding is used.

Since children with severe auditory processing problems need visual clues, I have devised a method of colour coding all the phonemes so that when making word lists and sentences for practice in workbooks, each phoneme to be learned is underlined once or twice, depending on whether the phoneme is voiceless or voiced.

Each pair of phonemes has an individual colour. A regular packet of 12 colours and one grey lead is enough.

The colour in which the written letters are underlined represents the SOUND those letters make regardless of how the word is spelt. Therefore, the word 'faces' would be written like this:

$$f a c e s$$

The children are quick to learn that each colour represents a sound. The colour coding is an integral part of the system and should be regarded as importantly as the hand cues. The colour coding is very useful in that the actual printed word never has to be changed.

The twenty-six consonant sounds are colour coded as follows:

one orange line	/ p /	/ b /	two orange lines
one pale blue line	/ t /	/ d /	two pale blue lines
one brown line	/ k /	/ g /	two brown lines
one orange line and one black line	/ m /	/ n /	one pale blue line and one black line
one brown line and one black line	/ ŋ /	/ h /	one grey pencil line
one pink line	/ f /	/ v /	two pink lines
one pale green line	/ s /	/ z /	two pale green lines
one red line	/ ʃ /	/ ʒ /	two red lines
one dark blue line	/ θ /	/ ð /	two dark blue lines
one purple line	/ tʃ /	/ dʒ /	two purple lines
two yellow lines	/ l /	/ r /*	two dark green lines
small red circle to suggest lip rounding	/ w /*	/ j /*	small red oval to suggest lip spreading
small red circle and grey pencil line	/ ʍ /	/ ç /	small red oval and grey pencil line

* **Note:** Do not colour code / r /, / w / and / j / when they are being used as vowels—only when they represent a consonant sound.

You will notice that all the phonemes where the lips are involved are coloured with pinks, reds, and oranges, (lipstick colours!). I always talk about snakes and blue-tongued lizards to the children to help them connect the sounds for blues and greens, i.e. the tongue sounds. / h / is grey because it is a 'misty' sort of sound—the colour of the vapour that is blown from the mouth on a cold day. I have always used brown for / k / and / g /, and / l / is yellow, because so many children call 'yellow' 'lellow' so it always seems appropriate to colour / l / yellow. / tʃ / and / dʒ / are purple because blue and red together make purple and / t / (blue) and / ʃ / (red) make / tʃ / (purple).

I have found colour coding very helpful indeed, but it must be used consistently and correctly. English spelling is very quirky but if the colour coding is used it helps with pronunciation. It is particularly useful when teaching English as a second language and to the hearing impaired.

Consonant table

In each column, voiceless consonants are on the left, and voiced consonants are on the right	Bi-labial (both lips)	Labio-dental (lips and teeth)	Dental (teeth)	Alveolar (teeth ridge)	Palato-alveolar	Palatal (hard palate)	Velar (soft palate)	Glottal (glottis)
Plosive	/p/ /b/			/t/ /d/			/k/ /g/	
Fricative/ Continuant	/ʍ/	/f/ /v/	/θ/ /ð/	/s/ /z/ /r/	/ʃ/ /ʒ/	/ç/		/h/
Affricate					/tʃ/ /dʒ/			
Nasal	/m/			/n/			/ŋ/	
Lateral				/l/				
Semivowel	/w/					/j/		

7

List of consonants

Consonant sound	Page
/ p /	10
/ b /	11
/ t /	12
/ d /	13
/ k /	14
/ g /	15
/ m /	16
/ n /	17
/ ŋ /	18
/ h /	19
/ f /	20
/ v /	21
/ s /	22
/ z /	23
/ ʃ /	24
/ ʒ /	25
/ θ /	26
/ ð /	27
/ tʃ /	28
/ dʒ /	29
/ l /	30
/ r /	31
/ w /	32
/ j /	34
/ ʍ /	36
/ ç /	36

/p / as in pick. Voiceless bi-labial plosive.

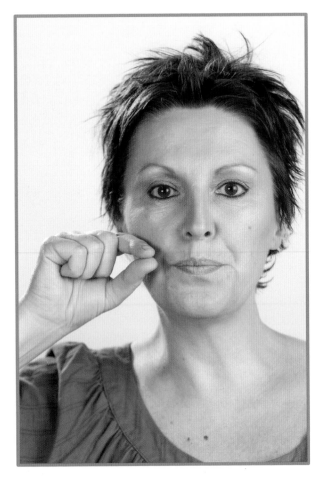

The picture depicts the starting point of the pronunciation of the phoneme / p /. As the lips separate to release the air the index finger separates from the thumb.

The shape of the hand with the index finger closed on the thumb suggests the way the lips must be for the production of this sound. The position of the fingers next to the lips, indicates where the sound is made. The movement of the finger and thumb separating shows what the lips must do to produce this sound.

/b̲ / as in b̲all. Voiced bi-labial plosive.

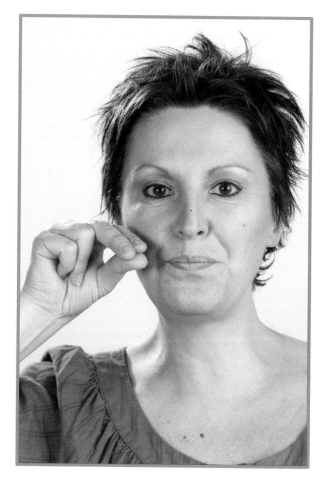

The picture depicts the starting point of the pronunciation of the phoneme / b̲ /.
As the lips separate to release the air the fingers separate from the thumb.

/ t / as in top. Voiceless alveolar plosive.

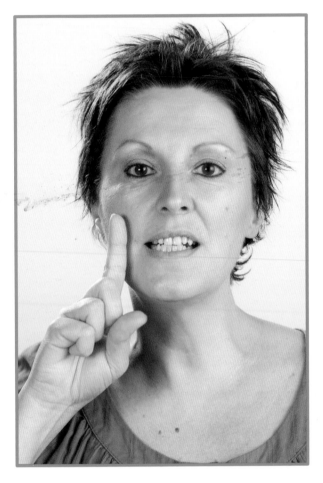

The picture depicts the start of the phoneme / t /. As the tongue releases the air stopped against the alveolar ridge to produce the phoneme / t /, the index finger is jerked forward approximately 2.5 centimetres (1 inch).

/ d̲ / as in d̲oor. Voiced alveolar plosive.

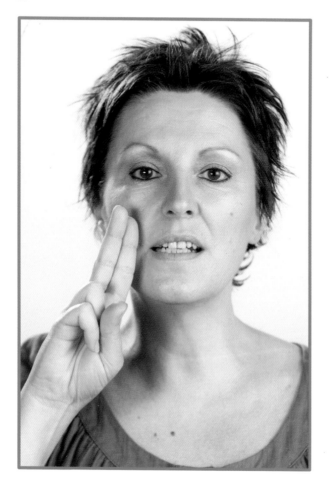

The picture depicts the start of the phoneme / d̲ /. As the tongue releases the air stopped against the alveolar ridge to produce the / d̲ / phoneme, the index and second fingers are jerked forward approximately 2.5 centimetres (1 inch).

/ k̲ / as in k̲ing. Voiceless velar plosive.

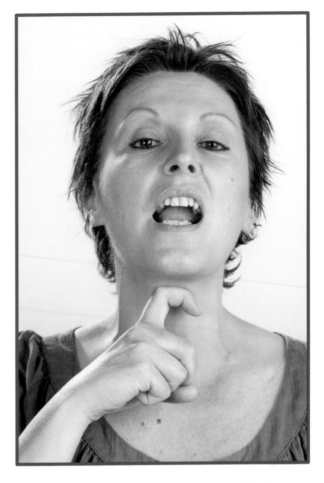

The picture depicts the starting point of the phoneme / k̲ /. As the air, which is stopped between the raised back of the tongue and the back of the palate, is released on the production of the phoneme / k̲ /, the crooked finger is jerked downwards and forward approximately 2.5 centimetres (1 inch).

/g/ as in go. Voiced velar plosive.

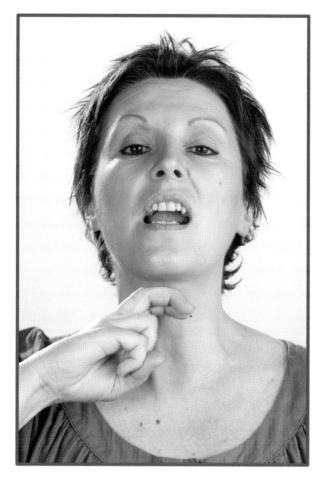

As for /k/ but with index and second finger crooked.

/ m̱ / as in m̱y. Voiced bi-labial nasal.

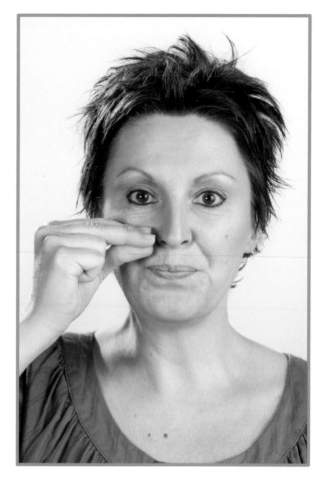

The hand is in the same shape as for / ḇ / but the fingers and thumb are placed on the side of the nose. The hand does not move on production of the phoneme.

In the production of / m̱ / the soft palate is lowered to allow the sound to come down the nose. The / m̱ / sound in fact is a nasal / ḇ /, and the hand sign indicates this.

/ n / as in no. Voiced alveolar nasal.

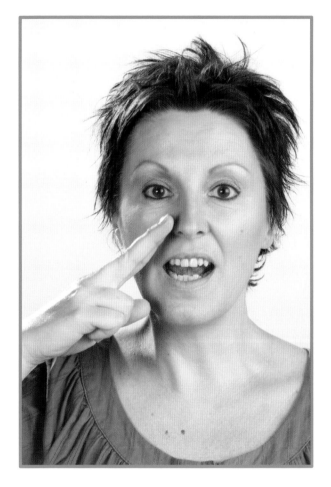

The hand is in the same shape as for / d / but the fingers are placed on the side of the nose. The hand does not move in the production of the phoneme.

In the production of / n / the soft palate is lowered to allow the sounds to come down the nose. The / n / is a nasal / d / and the hand sign indicates this.

/ ŋ / as in ring. Voiced velar nasal.

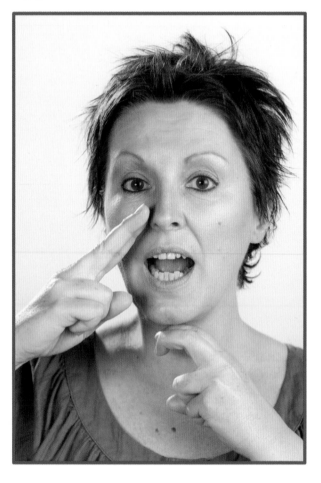

One hand as for / n / and the other as for / g / (this is the only two handed sign). The hands do not move during the production of the phoneme.

The sound is the one heard at the end of the word 'sing'—it is often confused with the / n / sound. It never occurs in an initial position in English. It is in fact a nasal / g / and the hands clearly indicate this with one hand signing / n / and the other / g /.

/ h / as in hat. Voiceless glottal continuant.

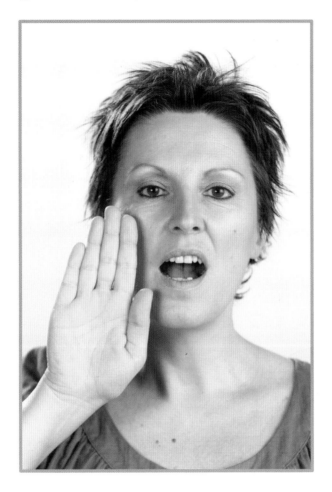

The hand is held as in the picture and indicates the glottis is open and the air is allowed to pass freely through the mouth without any obstruction. The hand is moved gently forward approximately 5 centimetres (2 inches) as the / h / is articulated to indicate that the air must continue through the mouth.

/ f / as in face. Voiceless labio-dental fricative.

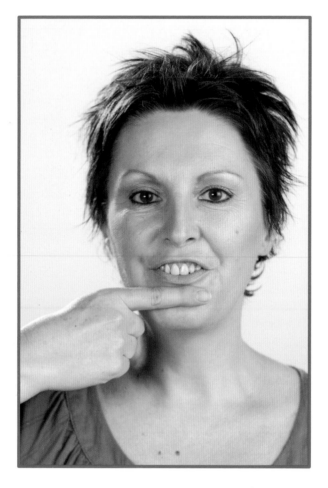

The picture depicts the starting point of the phoneme / f /. As the / f / is articulated, the shape of the hand remains the same but is moved downwards and forwards for approximately 10 centimetres (4 inches).

The movement of the hand shows the air is continuing out of the mouth to produce this sound. This is a very useful clue for the hearing impaired. / f / is often pronounced as a plosive or 'stop' sound. However well one lip-reads, one cannot see the air stream. The moving hand indicates this.

/ v / as in van. Voiced labio-dental fricative.

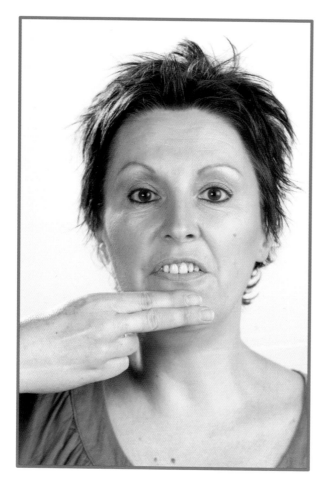

As for / f / but with second finger also extended.

/ s / as in sun. Voiceless alveolar fricative.

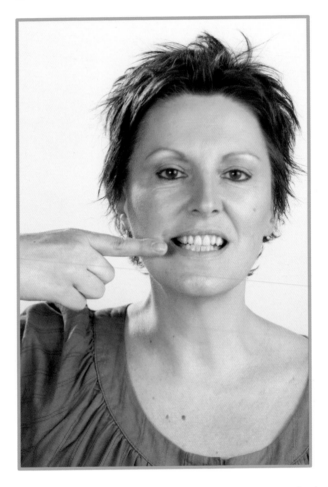

The picture depicts the start of the production of the phoneme / s /. As this sound is made, the shape of the hand remains the same but describes a wavy line in the air moving forward, like an 's' written on its side, approximately 10 centimetres long (4 inches).

/z/ as in zoo. Voiced alveolar fricative.

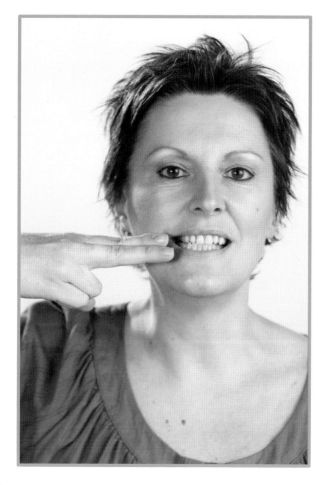

As for /s/, only two fingers are used and a zigzag line like a 'z' on its side is described moving forwards approximately 10 centimetres (4 inches).

/ ʃ / as in shine. Voiceless palato-alveolar fricative.

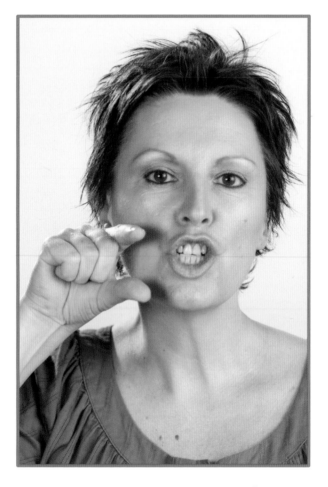

The picture depicts the starting point of the phoneme / ʃ /. The way in which the hand is held suggests the lip shape. As the / ʃ / phoneme is articulated the hand remains in this shape and moves straight forward approximately 10 centimetres (4 inches).

/ ʒ / as in measure. Voiced palato-alveolar fricative.

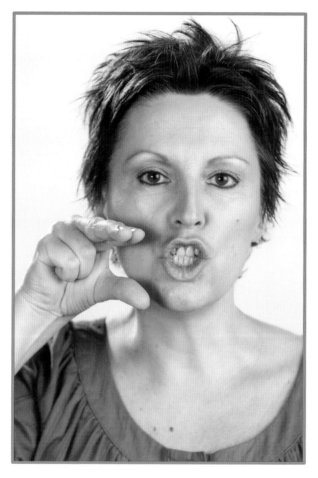

This phoneme is rarely used. It only appears in the middle of words like measure, pleasure and treasure but it is the voiced counterpart to the / ʃ / sound. There is no English grapheme to describe this sound. I have been able to teach profoundly deaf children how to make the / ʒ / sound by using this method. Make this phoneme the same way as / ʃ / but with two fingers extended as in the picture.

/ θ / as in think. Voiceless interdental fricative.

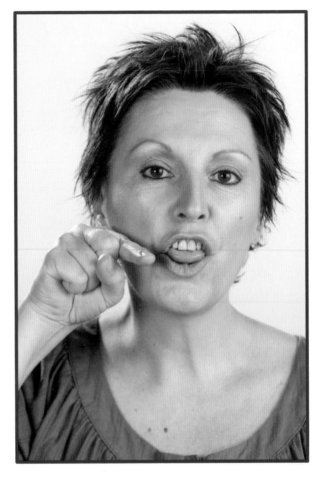

The picture indicates how the hand and tongue are placed at the start of the articulation of the phoneme / θ /. As the air escapes over the tongue, the hand is moved straight forward approximately 10 centimetres (4 inches). This phoneme is often mispronounced and teachers have found it useful to point out the differences in spelling between / f / for 'fin' and / θ / for 'thin'.

/ ð̬ / as in them. Voiced interdental fricative.

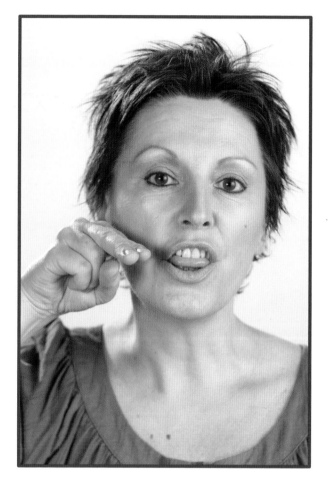

Move the hand in the same way as for / θ / but use two fingers to indicate that the sound is voiced.

In English both the 'th' in 'thin' and the 'th' in 'them' are written with the same two letters but they describe two different sounds; this is where the cues and the colour coding are so logical and helpful, as both show the voiced/voiceless contrast.

/ t∫ / as in <u>ch</u>ur<u>ch</u>. Voiceless palato-alveolar affricate.

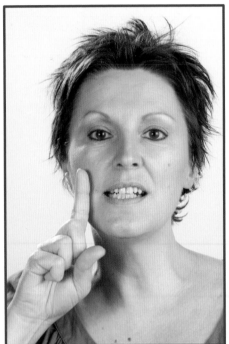 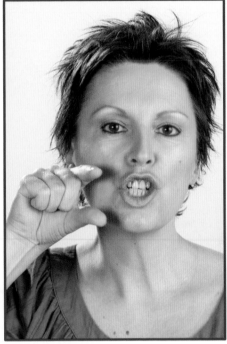

Sign <u>/ t /</u> and immediately afterwards drop the index finger down and bring the thumb forward and sign <u>/ ∫ /</u> moving the hand forward approximately 10 centimetres (4 inches).

/ dʒ / as in judge. Voiced palato-alveolar affricate.

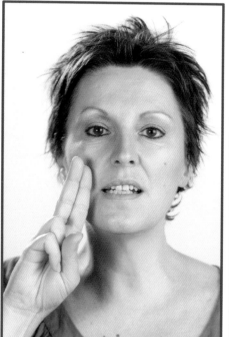 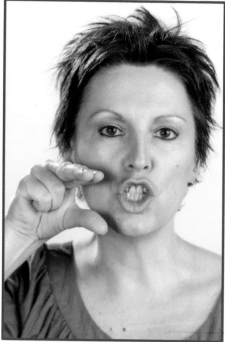

Sign / d / and immediately change hand sign to / ʒ / by dropping the two fingers down and bringing the thumb forward, then move the hand forward approximately 10 centimetres (4 inches).

/ l / as in lamp. Voiced alveloar lateral.

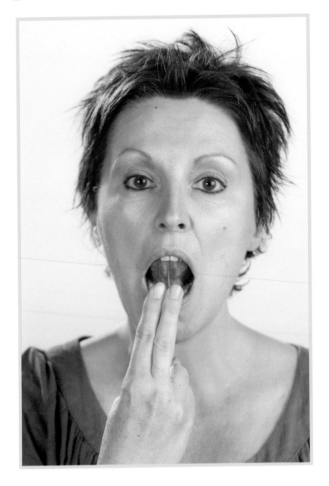

The picture indicates the way the hand is held for the start of the production of the / l / phoneme. Sometimes this phoneme is very difficult to produce and the fingers actually assist with pushing the tongue back and up. As the tongue glides or flaps to produce the / l / phoneme, the fingers describe a small semicircle downwards by action of the wrist.

/ r / as in run. Voiced retroflux fricative.

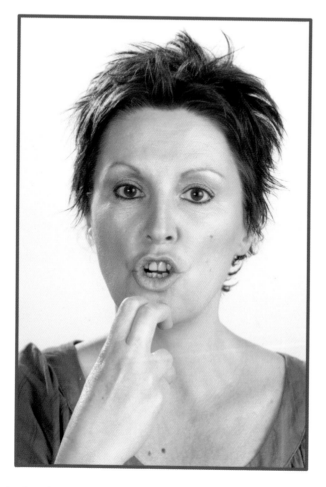

The picture depicts how the hand and mouth are held on production of the / r / phoneme. The shape of the fingers suggests the curled back movement of the tongue needed to produce this sound. The hand is only moved very slightly forwards and downwards by wrist action as the tongue articulates the / r / phoneme.

In Standard English the sound / r / is a rubbing sound made by the tongue tip curling up and slightly back to engage with the hard palate. This is the sound we hear at the beginning of words like 'rose', 'wrong' and 'right'. The 'r' at the end of 'roar' is not pronounced in the same way as the initial / r / sound—it becomes part of the vowel.

/ w / as in way. Voiced rounded semivowel.

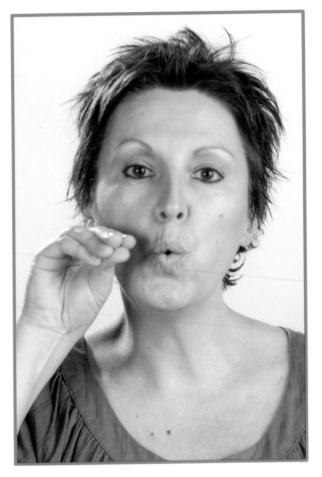

A

This phoneme is a semivowel, i.e. at the beginning of words it is used as a consonant but at the end of the word (such as in 'cow') it turns into a vowel. Two pictures are needed to describe the production of this phoneme. Picture A shows the hand shape suggesting rounded lips for the start of the production of / w /.

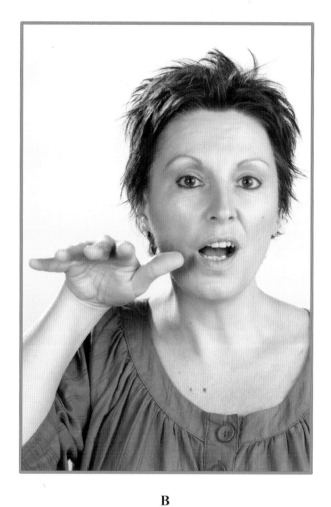

B

Picture B shows the fingers separated and the lips parted as the / w / sound is completed.

The small red circle under the / w / is only used when the / w / is used as a consonant, i.e. at the beginning of a word. It serves as a reminder that the lips must be rounded to produce the / w / phoneme.

/ j / as in yacht. Voiced spread semivowel.

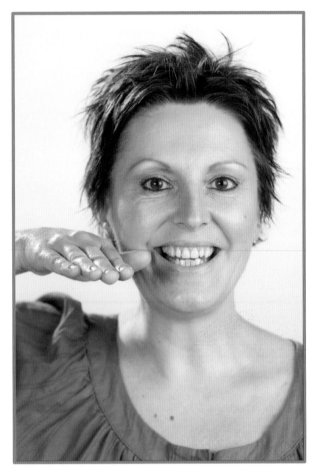

A

This is also a semivowel in that it has a double function, being used as a consonant at the beginning of words and a vowel at the end. These pictures describe the / j / when it is used as a consonant. Picture A shows how the hand and lips are held at the start of the production of the phenome / j /. The flat hand with fingers pointing forwards suggests the spread lips and raised tongue.

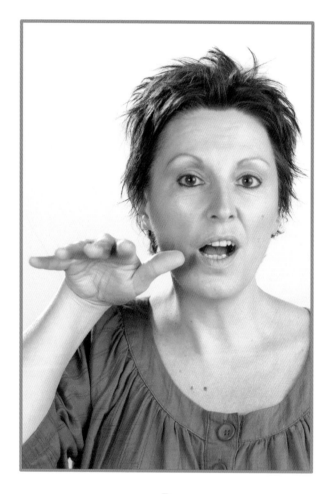

B

In picture B the fingers are spread and the lips slightly parted at the end of the production of the / j / phoneme.

The oval shape written under the / j / phoneme suggests the lips must be spread to produce a correct / j / sound. The initial / j / in 'yet', 'yes' and 'yak' would have the red oval under it, but not the 'y' at the end of the word where the letter serves to make a vowel (as in 'say') or where the 'y' can actually act as a vowel sound as in the word 'bossy'.

/ ʍ / as in white. Voiceless bi-labial continuant.

This sound is the voiceless pair to the semivowel / w /.

This is the initial sound in the words 'why', 'what', 'where', 'whip', etc. Many people do not make the distinction between / w / and / ʍ / and pronounce the sound as the semivowel / w /.

Sign / h / and immediately after sign / w / and blend the sounds together as you sign and say them.

/ ç / as in human. Voiceless palatal fricative.

This sound is the voiceless pair to the semivowel / j /.

It is the initial sound in the words 'human', 'hue', 'humid', 'Hugh', 'huge', etc. There are not very many words in English that start with this sound, and there is only one written symbol to describe two different sounds. The 'h' at the beginning of 'happy' sounds different to the 'h' at the beginning of 'huge'. This is where the colour coding really helps.

Sign / h / and immediately after sign / j / and blend the sounds together as you sign and say them.

The vowels

Vowels are notoriously difficult to establish and correct if one does not acquire them naturally; perhaps this is because they have to be recognised by the ear. They cannot be described in print as easily as consonants. With vowels the variation between sounds has to be heard to be fully appreciated and understood. Also, we only have five written symbols to describe twenty-three sounds.

The hand signs I have devised to represent the vowel sounds are—as indeed the consonants are—based on where they are made in the mouth, whether there is lip rounding or not, and also whether they are long vowels, short vowels, diphthongs or triphthongs. It is hoped that the hand signs will serve to remind people who have problems with the pronunciation of vowels how to make them successfully.

Vowels are sounds made by allowing the breath to pass freely through the mouth. The tongue and lips alter their positions for every vowel, but do not move sufficiently near to any part of the mouth to check the flow of breath. Vowels are always voiced—the vocal cords must vibrate to produce them—the tip of the tongue should be in contact with the lower teeth when any vowel is being produced. This is important as it counteracts the tendency to retract the tongue. Please refer to the organs of speech diagram on p. 39 to see these parts of the mouth illustrated.

Out of the large number of vowel sounds used by English-speaking people, a set of twelve pure vowels, nine diphthongs and two triphthongs have been selected. This set of sounds represents the type of pronunciation accepted by most listeners as representing Standard English. Probably there are very few speakers who are exact in their use of this set of sounds, but provided there is a fairly close approximation to them, slight variations are not important. It is the acceptance of this particular set of sounds by speakers of widely varying types of English which gives it value as a standard.

It would be too cumbersome and confusing to colour code each vowel separately, but sometimes it is useful to put a red DOT above the short vowels, and a red LINE above the long vowels as shown on the cards and posters available from ACER Press.

The lips should be spread in varying degrees for all the front vowels. These vowels are called front vowels because the front of the tongue moves to adjust the shape of the mouth resonator. (Remember the tip of the tongue is anchored behind the lower teeth for all vowel sounds.)

The lips should be rounded in varying degrees for all the back vowels. For the back vowels the back of the tongue moves to adjust the shape of the mouth resonator.

There are three central vowels, where the centre of the tongue moves to adjust the shape of the mouth resonator. The lips are in a more-or-less neutral position for these sounds and are neither spread nor rounded to any degree.

Diphthongs

A diphthong is a glide sound. The tongue starts in the position for one sound and moves immediately towards another vowel position. All the diphthongs in English are falling diphthongs, that is to say, the impulse is strong on the first element and weak on the second.

Triphthongs

There are two triphthongs. These sounds are considered as one syllable, but three distinct sounds should be heard. Often the first element of diphthongs and triphthongs are stressed and the second and third elements are weakened so that they practically disappear. Care must be taken to pronounce each element clearly and glide smoothly between them—the hand signs will help with this.

Organs of speech

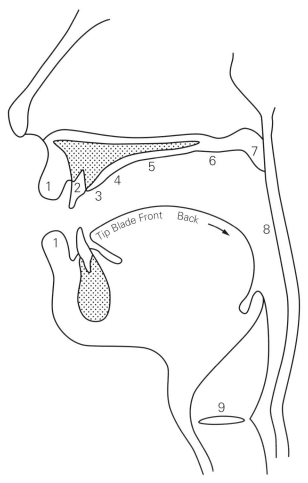

1. Lips (labial)
2. Teeth (dental)
3. Alveolar ridge (alveolar)
4. Hard palate (pre-palatal)
5. Hard palate (palatal)
6. Soft palate (velar)
7. Uvula (uvular)
8. Pharynx (pharyngeal)
9. Glottis (glottal)

The vowel sounds of Standard English

Pure Vowels					
1.	/ i /	eve	beat	*Front vowels*	Lips spread in varying degrees for front vowels
2.	/ ɪ /	in	bit		
3.	/ ɛ /	end	bet		
4.	/ æ /	at	bat		
5.	/ a /	arm	car	*Back vowels*	Lips rounded in varying degrees for back vowels
6.	/ ɒ /	on	not		
7.	/ ɔ /	or	bought		
8.	/ ʊ /		put		
9.	/ u /	ooze	moon		
10.	/ ʌ /	up	bun	*Central vowels*	Lips in neutral state for central vowels
11.	/ ɜ /	earn	bird		
12.	/ ə /	about	around		

Diphthongs			
13.	/ ɛɪ /	aim	day
14.	/ əʊ /	owe	go
15.	/ aɪ /	eye	high
16.	/ aʊ /	out	now
17.	/ ɔɪ /	oil	boy
18.	/ ɪə /	ear	here
19.	/ ɛə /	air	there
20.	/ ɔə /		more
21.	/ ʊə /		poor

Triphthongs			
22.	/ aɪə /	ire	fire
23.	/ aʊə /	our	flower

Diagram 1

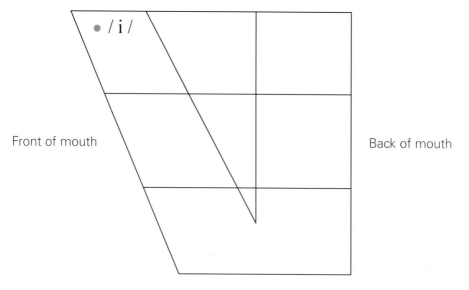

Diagram of mouth resonator showing placement of vowel / i /

Imagine this is the shape of the mouth resonator. The vowel / i / as in 'eat' is a 'close front vowel', which means the front of the tongue is placed at the front of the mouth (remember the tip of the tongue is anchored behind the lower teeth) and the air is restricted by the closeness of the tongue to the roof of the mouth. The dot indicates roughly where the front of the tongue should be placed for the production of this sound.

Diagram 2

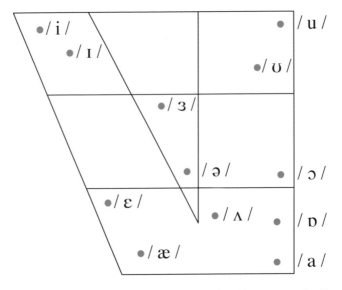

The placement of each vowel in the mouth can be diagrammatically shown.

Diagram 3

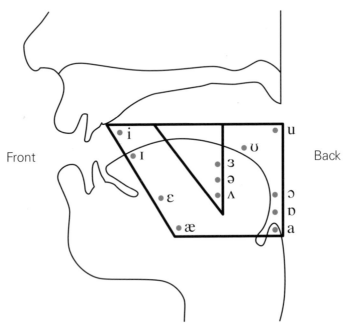

Each vowel is shown schematically in relation to the vertical and horizontal position of the arch of the tongue for its production.

List of vowels

Vowel number	Vowel sound	Page
1	/ i / (eve)	44
2	/ ɪ / (in)	46
3	/ ɛ / (egg)	48
4	/ æ / (apple)	50
5	/ a / (arm)	52
6	/ ɒ / (ox)	54
7	/ ɔ / (or)	56
8	/ ʊ / (book)	58
9	/ u / (ooze)	60
10	/ ʌ / (up)	62
11	/ ɜ / (earn)	64
12	/ ə / (about)	66
13	/ ɛɪ / (aim)	69
14	/ əʊ / (owe)	70
15	/ aɪ / (eye)	71
16	/ aʊ / (out)	72
17	/ ɔɪ / (oil)	73
18	/ ɪə / (ear)	74
19	/ ɛə / (air)	75
20	/ ɔə / (more)	76
21	/ ʊə / (poor)	77
22	/ aɪə / (ire)	78
23	/ aʊə / (our)	79

Vowel 1: / i / as in <u>e</u>ve.

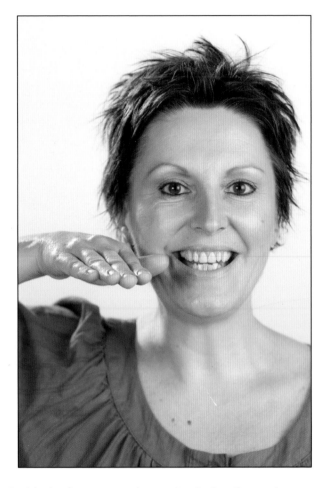

The flat hand with the fingers together and pointing forwards suggests the raised tongue and spread lips. Since this is a long vowel, the hand is moved forward 10 centimetres, or approximately one hand's length, when the vowel is articulated.

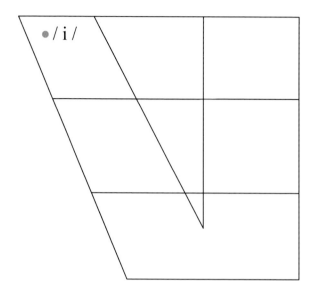

Description

Tongue: Tip is behind lower teeth.
Front is raised towards hard palate.
Sides are raised to sides of upper teeth.

Lips: Spread.

Teeth: Slightly apart.

Words containing / i / sound: eve, meat, mete, receive, siege, key, quay.

Vowel 2: / ɪ / as in in.

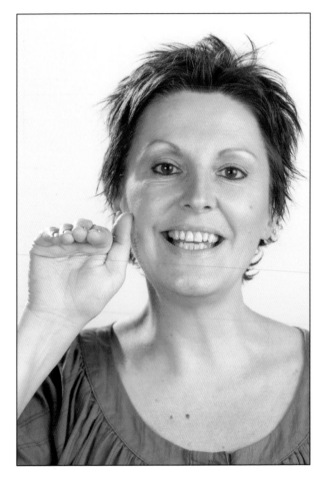

The hand sign shows the position of the tongue in the mouth. As the / ɪ / sound is articulated, the hand should be jerked forward very slightly to show it is a short vowel—as if the fingers were 'dotting the i'.

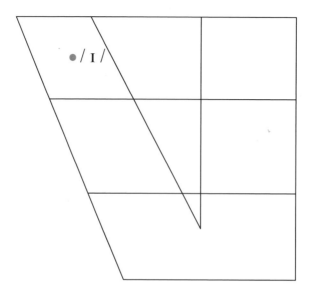

Description

Tongue: Almost the same as / i /, but the front of the tongue is not raised so far towards the hard palate. The tip and sides of the tongue are in the same position as / i /.

Lips: Half spread.

Teeth: Slightly apart.

Words containing / ɪ / sound: in<u>ci</u>v<u>i</u>l<u>i</u>ty, b<u>u</u>sy, s<u>ie</u>ve, forf<u>ei</u>t, b<u>i</u>sc<u>ui</u>t.

Vowel 3: / ɛ / as in <u>e</u>gg.

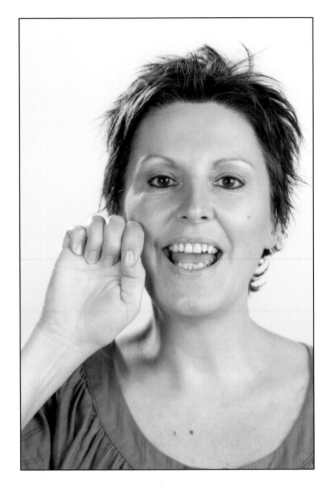

The hand sign suggests the position of the tongue in the mouth. As the / ɛ / sound is articulated, the hand should be jerked forward very slightly to show it is a short vowel.

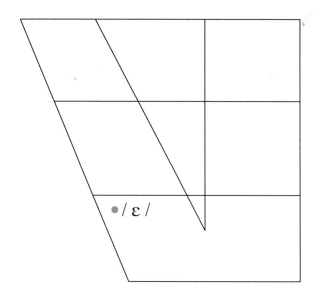

Description

Tongue: Front of the tongue is raised towards hard palate but not as humped as for / ɪ /.

Lips: In a normal neutral position.

Jaw: Slightly lowered.

Words containing / ɛ / sound: end, engine, friend, get, bury, many, leopard, said, guess, head.

Vowel 4: / æ / as in apple.

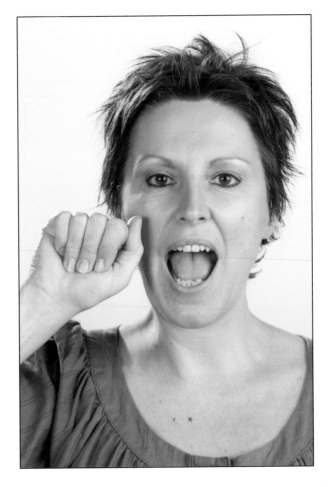

The hand sign suggests the shape of the mouth. I usually compare this sound with the word apple and suggest the hand looks like an apple. The hand is jerked forward slightly indicating a short vowel.

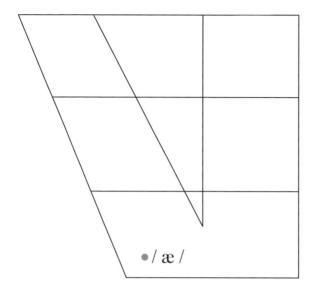

/ æ /

Description

Tongue: Front of the tongue is slightly raised.

Lips: Slightly drawn back.

Jaw: Slightly lower than for / ɛ /.

Words containing / æ / sound: <u>a</u>nt, b<u>a</u>t, pl<u>ai</u>d, h<u>a</u>ve.

Vowel 5: / a / as in a<u>r</u>m.

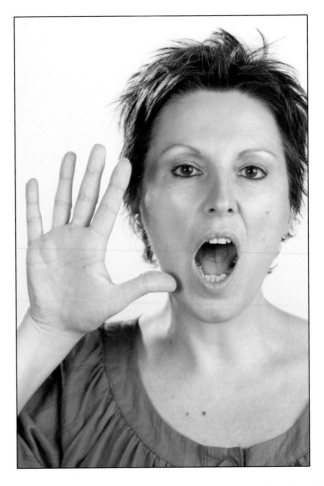

The hand sign suggests the open mouth. The movement of the hand backwards (approximately 10 centimetres or 4 inches) shows that it is a long sound. The movement backwards shows the vowel is made at the back of the mouth.

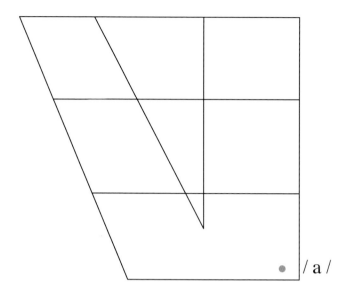

/ a /

Description

Tongue: The back of the tongue is slightly raised but the tongue is low in the mouth.

Lips: More rounded than for / æ / and more relaxed.

Jaw: Well dropped.

Words containing / a / sound: arm, aunt, calm, clerk, heart, guard, bazaar, park, laugh, grass.

Vowel 6: / ɒ / as in <u>o</u>x.

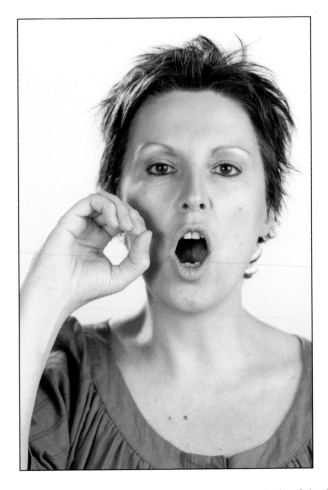

The hand sign suggests the rounding of the lips. A slight jerk of the hand backwards shows that it is a short back vowel.

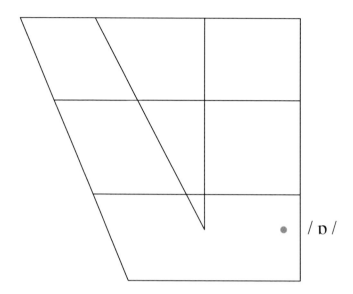

/ ɒ /

Description

Tongue: Back of the tongue is raised slightly towards the soft palate, but the tongue is low in the mouth.

Lips: Rounded, but relaxed.

Jaw: Dropped.

Words containing / ɒ / sound: <u>o</u>x, <u>o</u>range, w<u>a</u>nt, c<u>ou</u>gh, qu<u>a</u>lity, y<u>a</u>cht, t<u>o</u>p.

Vowel 7: / ɔ / as in <u>or</u>.

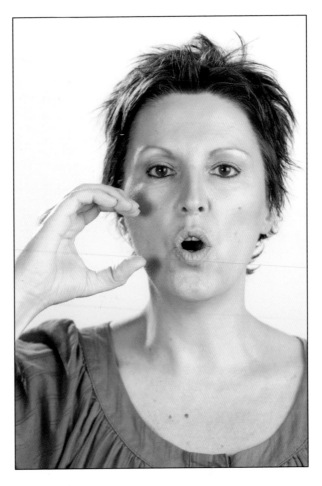

The hand sign suggests the rounding of the lips and the movement of the hand backwards approximately 10 centimetres or 4 inches shows it is a long sound.

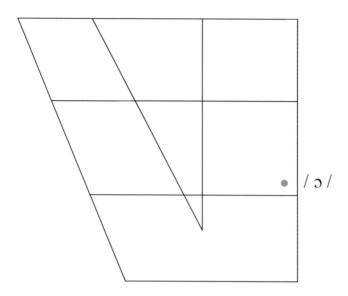

/ ɔ /

Description

Tongue: The back and middle of the tongue is raised towards the soft palate and hard palate, slightly further than for / ɒ /.

Lips: Rounded and pushed forward, the edges of the lips slightly forward.

Jaw: Dropped about the same amount as for / ɒ /.

Words containing / ɔ / sound: a̲w̲ful, fa̲ll, fo̲r, Pa̲u̲l, wa̲ter, co̲re, pa̲w̲, ta̲u̲ght.

Vowel 8: / ʊ / as in b<u>oo</u>k.

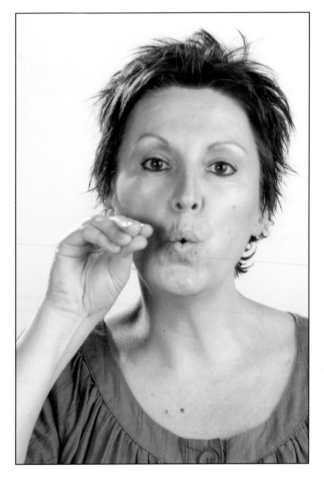

The hand sign suggests the close rounding of the lips, the slight jerk backwards on production tells us that the vowel is a short back sound.

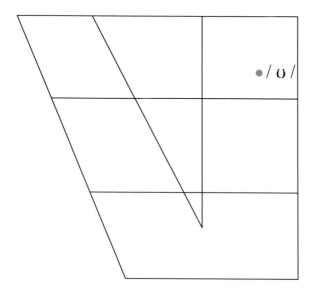

Description

Tongue: Back of the tongue is well raised towards soft palate.

Lips: Pushed forward and rounded.

Jaw: In a neutral position.

Words containing / ʊ / sound: b<u>oo</u>k, g<u>oo</u>d, w<u>ou</u>ld, f<u>u</u>ll.

Vowel 9: / u / as in <u>oo</u>ze.

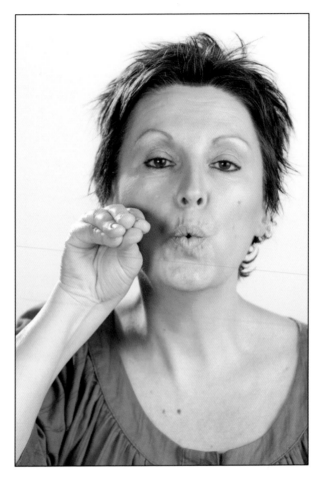

The hand sign suggests the close rounding of the lips and the movement of the hand backwards (approximately 10 centimetres or 4 inches) shows that it is made at the back of the mouth and that it is a long vowel.

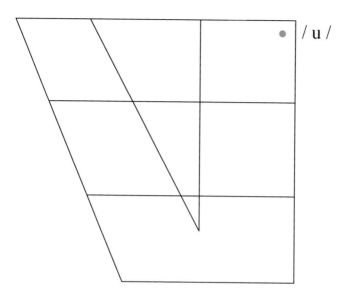

/ u /

Description

Tongue: The back of the tongue is raised close to the soft palate.

Lips: Close rounded and pushed forward vigorously.

Jaw: In a neutral position.

Words containing / u / sound: wh<u>o</u>se, pr<u>u</u>ne, sh<u>oe</u>, thr<u>ough</u>, t<u>wo</u>, t<u>oo</u>, t<u>o</u>.

Vowel 10: / ʌ / as in u̲p.

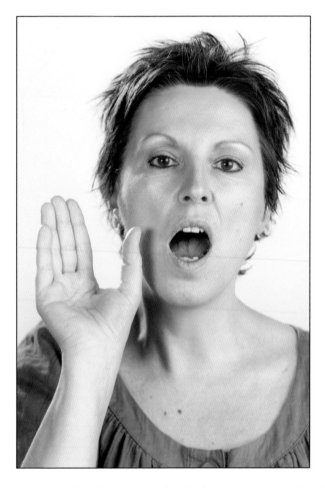

The hand sign suggests the shape of the initial letter in the word 'up' and the slight jerk outwards on production shows it is a short central vowel.

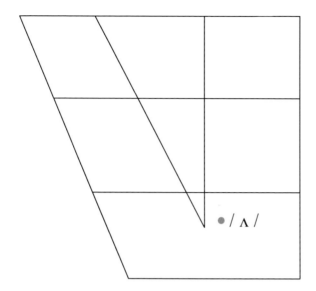

Description

Tongue: There is a slight raising of the tongue at a point between the centre and back towards the hard palate.

Lips: In a natural, slightly open relaxed position.

Jaw: In a neutral position.

Words containing / ʌ / sound: b<u>u</u>t, l<u>o</u>ve, bl<u>oo</u>d, r<u>ou</u>gh, <u>o</u>ne, d<u>oe</u>s.

Vowel 11: / 3 / as in <u>ear</u>n.

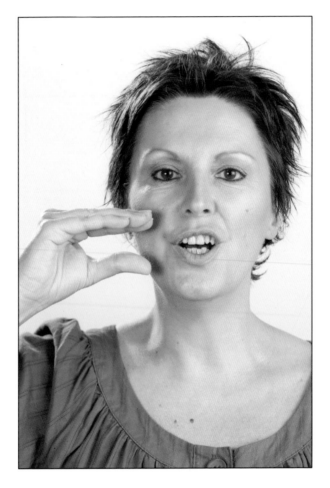

The hand sign suggests the slight spreading of the lips. The movement of the hand outwards (approximately 10 centimetres or 4 inches) shows it is a long central vowel.

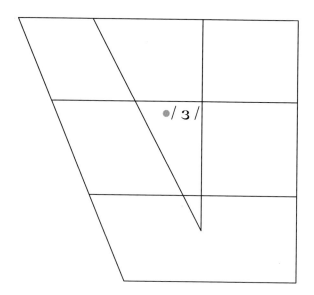

Description

Tongue: Raised at the centre.

Lips: In neutral slightly spread position.

Jaw: In a neutral position.

This is a long vowel, not to be confused with / ʌ / which is a short vowel.

Words containing / ɜ / sound: b<u>ir</u>d, t<u>er</u>m, sk<u>ir</u>t, l<u>ear</u>n, w<u>or</u>ld, f<u>ur</u>.

Vowel 12: / ə / as in about.

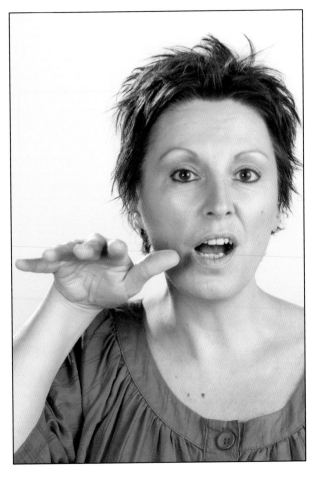

The hand sign is the same as for the second element of the semivowels / j / and / w / as described in the consonant section.

The hand should be held lightly, and the fingers jerked outwards slightly as the vowel is said.

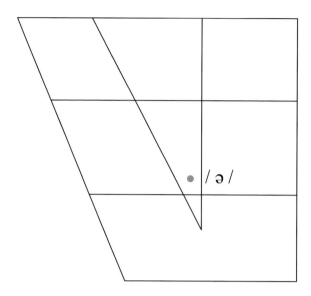

Description

Tongue: The middle of the tongue is nearly flat.

Lips: In a neutral position.

Jaw: In a neutral position.

This sound is the most frequently used in spoken English. It is often called the 'schwa' sound.

Words containing / ə / sound: th<u>e</u> (before consonants), <u>a</u>bove, bett<u>er</u>, mart<u>yr</u>, sof<u>a</u>, <u>a</u> (as in 'a stone').

Diphthongs

A diphthong is a glide sound. The tongue starts in the position for one vowel sound and moves immediately towards another vowel position. It does not necessarily reach it. It is important to make the glide smoothly and quickly, and without stopping between the two elements.

The Standard English diphthongs are all known as falling diphthongs. The emphasis is strong on the first element and weak on the second.

Vowel 13: / ɛɪ / as in a<u>i</u>m.

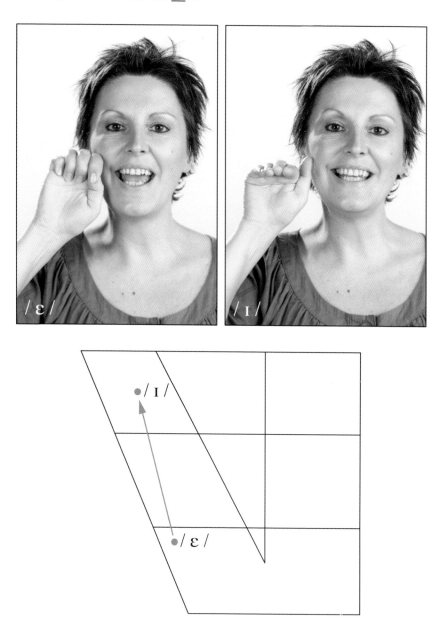

Sign / ɛ / and then / ɪ /.

Words containing / ɛɪ / diphthong: v<u>ei</u>n, d<u>ay</u>, th<u>ey</u>, fl<u>a</u>me, gr<u>ea</u>t, p<u>ai</u>d, g<u>au</u>ge.

Vowel 14: / əʊ / as in <u>owe</u>.

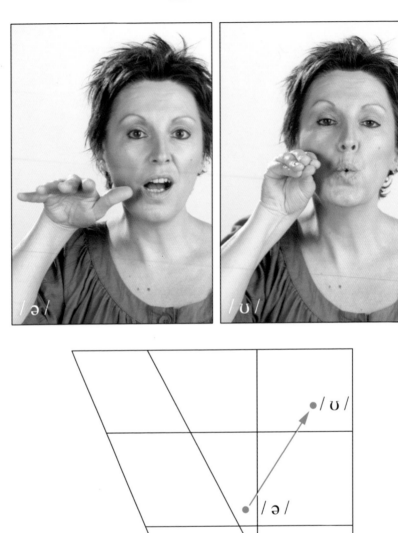

Sign / ə / and then / ʊ /.

Words containing the / əʊ / diphthong: s<u>o</u>, s<u>ew</u>, kn<u>ow</u>, c<u>oc</u><u>oa</u>, br<u>oo</u>ch, h<u>oe</u>, d<u>ou</u>gh, <u>oh</u>, m<u>au</u>ve.

Vowel 15: / aɪ / as in <u>eye</u>.

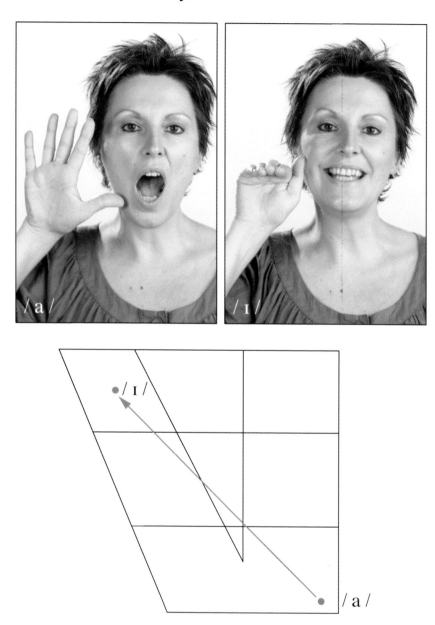

Sign / a / and then / ɪ /.

Words containing the / aɪ / diphthong: <u>I</u>, <u>eye</u>, b<u>y</u>, b<u>uy</u>, l<u>i</u>ght, <u>ai</u>sle, <u>ay</u>e, g<u>ui</u>de, p<u>ie</u>, h<u>ei</u>ght, d<u>ie</u>d, r<u>i</u>de.

Vowel 16: / aʊ / as in <u>out</u>.

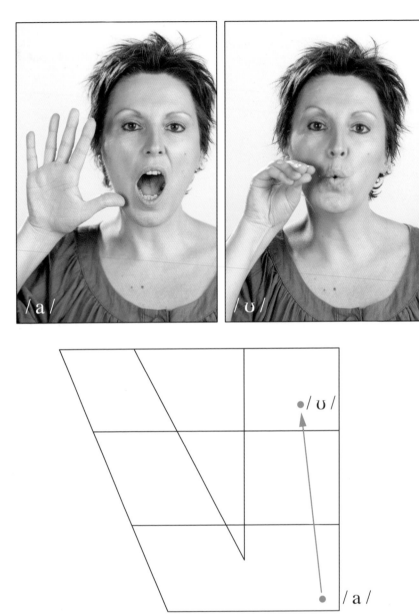

Sign / a / and then / ʊ /.

Words containing the / aʊ / diphthong: <u>ou</u>t, c<u>ow</u>, b<u>ough</u>, th<u>ou</u>.

Vowel 17: / ɔɪ / as in <u>oi</u>l.

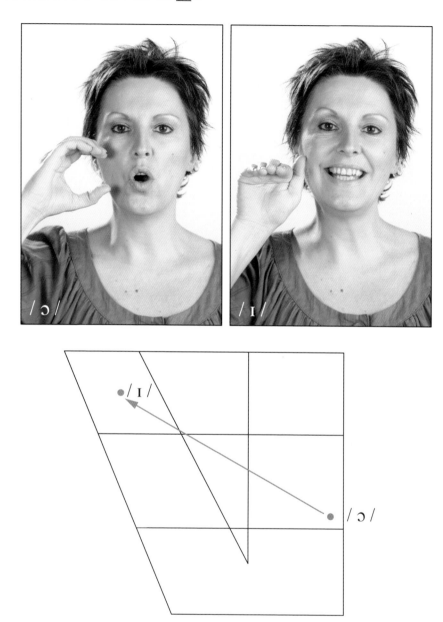

Sign / ɔ / and then / ɪ /.

Words containing the / ɔɪ / diphthong: b<u>oy</u>, b<u>oi</u>l, b<u>uoy</u>.

Vowel 18: / ɪə / as in <u>ear</u>.

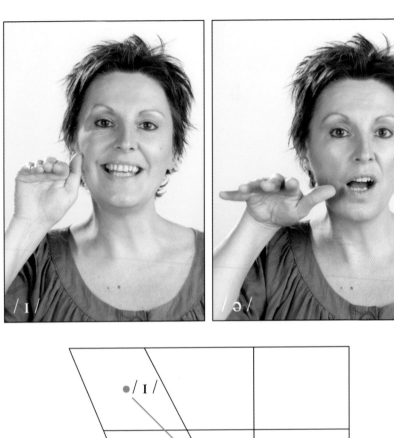

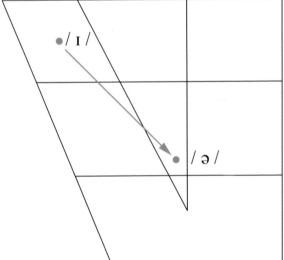

Sign / ɪ / and then / ə /.

Words containing the / ɪə / diphthong: s<u>ea</u>r, b<u>ee</u>r, b<u>ie</u>r, b<u>ea</u>rd, w<u>ei</u>r.

Vowel 19: / ɛə / as in <u>air</u>.

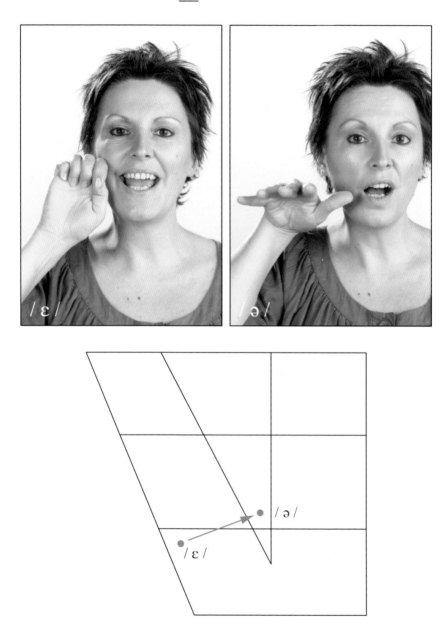

Sign / ɛ / and then / ə /.

Words containing the / ɛə / diphthong: wh<u>ere</u>, p<u>air</u>, th<u>eir</u>, fl<u>are</u>, m<u>ayor</u>, pr<u>ayer</u>.

Vowel 20: / ɔə / as in m<u>ore</u>.

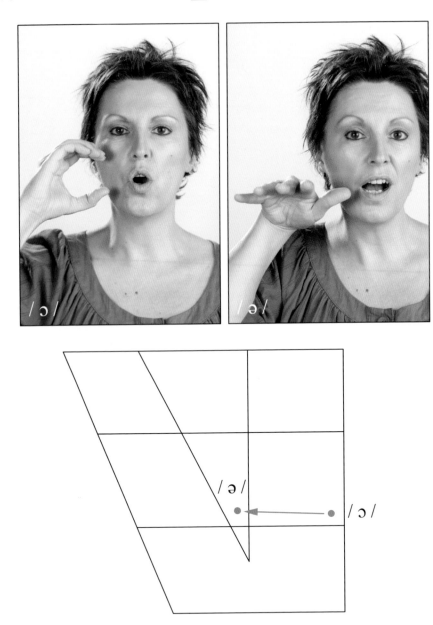

Sign / ɔ / and then / ə /.

Words containing the / ɔə / diphthong: m<u>ore</u>, dr<u>awer</u>, d<u>oor</u>.

Vowel 21: / ʊə / as in p<u>oor</u>.

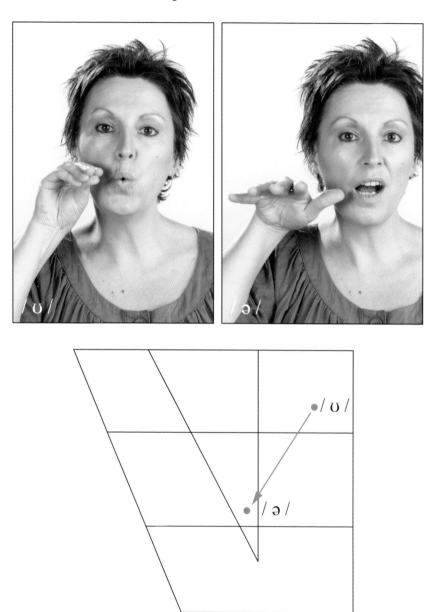

Sign / ʊ / and then / ə /.

Words containing the / ʊə / diphthong: p<u>oor</u>, t<u>our</u>, s<u>ure</u>.

Triphthongs

Vowel 22: / aɪə / as in <u>ire</u>.

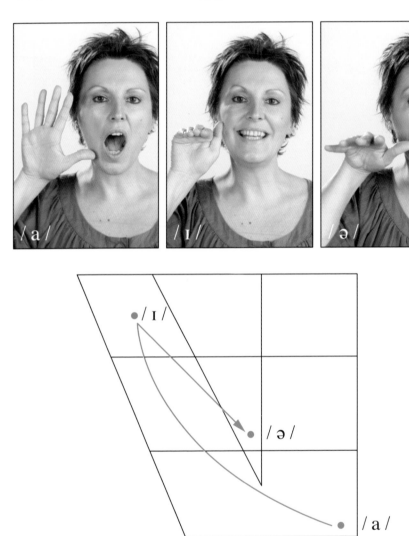

Sign / a / then / ɪ / and then / ə /.

Words containing / aɪə / triphthong: f<u>ire</u>, l<u>iar</u>, h<u>igher</u>, ch<u>oir</u>.

Vowel 23: / aʊə / as in <u>our</u>.

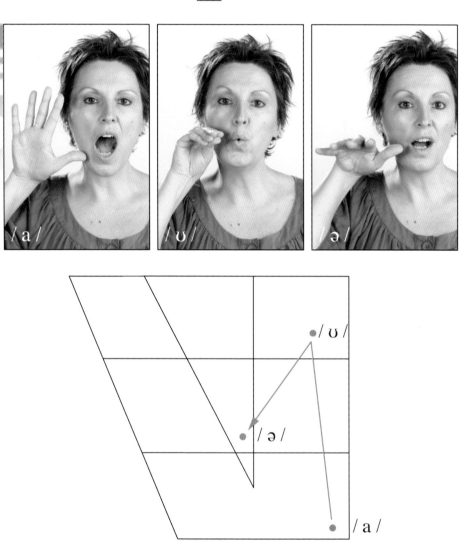

Sign / a / then / ʊ / and then / ə /.

Words containing / aʊə / triphthong: p<u>ower</u>, h<u>our</u>.

A family of resources availabl

Cued Articulation Consonants Posters - set of 2

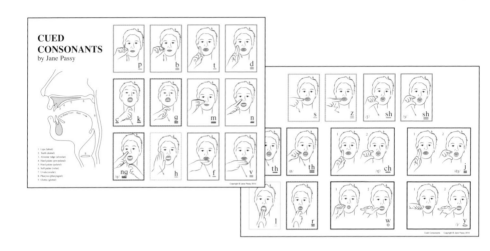

Cued Articulation Vowels Posters - set of 2

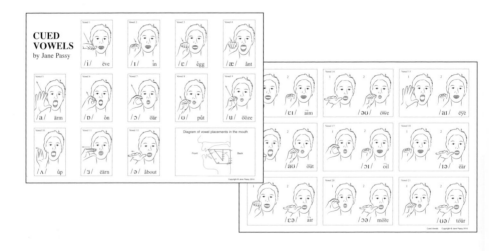

Visit http://shop.acer.edu.au

r use with Cued Articulation

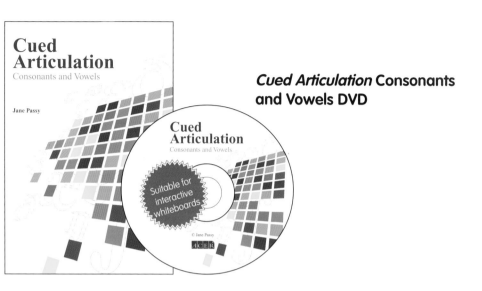

Cued Articulation Consonants and Vowels DVD

Cued Articulation Vowels and Consonants Cards - set of 45

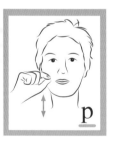

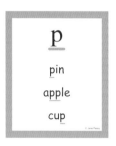

p

pin

apple

cup

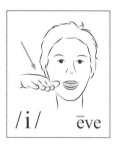

Vowel 1

/ i /

ēat

grēen

bēans

/ i /   ēve

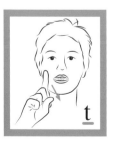

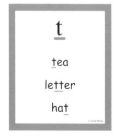

t

tea

letter

hat

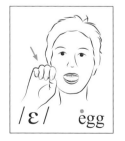

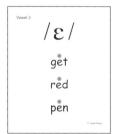

Vowel 3

/ ɛ /

gĕt

rĕd

pĕn

/ ɛ /   ĕgg

Visit http://shop.acer.edu.au

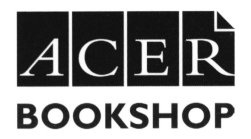

BOOKSHOP

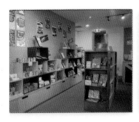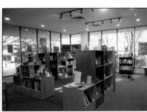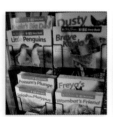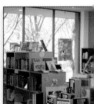

The ACER Bookshop specialises in:

- » Teacher Resources
- » Special Needs
- » Literacy
- » Numeracy
- » Speech and Language
- » Early Years

- » Student Wellbeing
- » Leadership and Management
- » Parenting
- » Study and Scholarship Materials
- » Research Publications

Ask our Bookseller to:

- » source publications for you from other publishers and distributors
- » quote and fulfill your entire school booklist
- » post your order to you, if necessary

MELBOURNE
19 Prospect Hill Road
Camberwell, Victoria
t: 03 9277 5490
h: Mon–Fri, 9am–5pm

BRISBANE
1/165 Kelvin Grove Road
Kelvin Grove, Queensland
t: 07 3238 9000
h: Mon–Fri, 9am–5pm

e: bookshop@acer.edu.au

PERTH
7/1329 Hay Street
West Perth, Western Austr
t: 08 9485 2194
h: Mon–Fri, 9am–5pm

www.acerbookshop.com.au

peech and Language Specialists

Articulation

Assessment

Auditory Processing

Basic Concepts

Grammar, Syntax and Literacy

Oral Motor, Voice and Fluency

Phonological Awareness

Social Skills

ralian Council *for* Educational Research

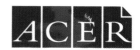